Respiratory Simulations

Student License and Workbook

Contributing Authors

Sherry Whiteman, MS, RRT
Missouri Southern State University

Caleb Lewis, BS, RRT
Missouri Southern State University

Janice Dunaway, MS, RRT
Missouri Southern State University

Glenda Pippin, BS, RRT, NPS, CPFT
Missouri Southern State University

Scot Jones, BA, RRT, ACCS
Broward College

Managing Editors

Dana Oakes, BA, RRT, NPS

Scot Jones, BA, RRT, ACCS
Broward College

Assisting Editors

Eric Dotten, MSL, REMT-P, NCEE
Broward College

Lezli Giancarlo, BS, RRT
Genesee Community College

Michael W. Hess, BS, RRT
U.S. Department of Verterans Affairs

Danielle Jones
Layout Assistant

Kathy S. Myers Moss, M.Ed., RRT, ACCS
University of Missouri

Monica Schibig, M.Ed., RRT
University of Missouri

Special Appreciation to

Broward College (especially the Health Sciences Simulation Center)
Genesee Community College
Missouri Southern State University

Printed in the United States of America.

ISBN 978-0-932887-50-4

RespiratoryBooks
A Division of Health Educator Publications, Inc.
4613 University Drive PMB 457
Coral Springs, Florida, USA

RespiratoryBooks.com

Attention:

This book serves as a User License for the 20 Adult Simulations contained within it. Health Educator Publications, Inc. issues the purchaser of this book ONE user license to participate in all 20 simulations for as long as you are part of the assigned course. This user license is non-transferable.

Your instructor will need the Performance Checklists prior to each simulaton, but will provide you instructions on when to provide these checklists. In addition, your instructor will assign "debrief assignments" for you following simulation experiences. Put your best into these - they will help shape who you are as a professional!

Simulations by Patient Name

Simulation Orientation Checklist		
Student Name:		
Date of Orientation:		
Area	**Skill**	**Initials Upon Completion**
Adult Manikin		
Head	Check pupils	
Neck	Check carotid pulse	
Chest	Attach leads (EKG/defib)	
	Auscultate all lung fields	
	Auscultate cardiac	
	Perform 5-10 chest compressions	
Abdomen	Auscultate bowel sounds	
	Check femoral pulses	
Arms	Check radial pulses	
	Check brachial pulses	
	Check manual blood pressure	
Legs	Check pedal pulses	
	Check posterior tibial pulse	
Neonate Manikin *(optional: for those participating in neonatal simulations)*		
Head	Inspect eyes	
	Inspect fontanel	
Chest	Attach leads (EKG/defib)	
	Auscultate breath sounds	
	Auscultate cardiac	
Arms	Check radial pulses	
	Check brachial pulses	
Umbilical	Identify vessels	
	Check pulse	

Area	Skill	Initials Upon Completion
Patient Monitor and Equipment		
Monitor	Start automatic blood pressure	
	Start $ETCO_2$ waveform	
	Start EKG rhythm	
	Place SpO_2 on manikin	
Equipment	Turn on and set up suction	
	Connect flowmeter to oxygen and run at 2 L/min (then turn off and disconnect)	
	Locate and press Code Blue button	
	Locate the drug dispensary system	
	Locate where equipment can be found	
	Order labs, CXR, 12-lead EKG	
Code Cart (Crash Cart)		
	Open each door and identify items	
	Turn defibrillator on and off	
	Check connections and adapters	
	Locate CPR board	
Patient Bed		
	Raise bed up and down	
	Place in Trendelenburg	
	Raise head of bed to 45 degrees	
	Put rail down and then back up	
	Pull CPR handle to lower head of bed	
	Unlock and lock bed	

I have reviewed the above steps with my Instructor, and I feel comfortable using the equipment respectfully and safely. I understand that the simulation environment should be treated exactly like I am at a clinical site, with the same seriousness and respect. If I have any questions about equipment use, or if anything appears to not be working correctly, I will notify one of my instructors immediately.

Student Signature: ______________________________

PERFORMANCE CHECKLIST

Student Name: ______________________ Date Performed: ______________________

Objectives	Pass		Needs Improvement
	Exceeds Standards	Meets Standards	Below Standards
General Objectives			
Performs hand hygiene at all appropriate intervention points	Intervenes and reminds others of need for PPE and hand hygiene	Washes hands prior to all contact points, including in between interventions	Fails to perform hand hygiene prior to patient contact or at any other intervention point
Introduces self to the patient and/or family professionally	Introduces self to patient and family, displays friendly, professional behavior at all times	Introduces self to patient and family in a professional manner	Fails to introduce self to patient and/or family, OR fails to introduce self professionally
Identifies the patient using a minimum of 2 patient identifiers	Identifies patient using 2 identifiers and explains reasoning to patient briefly	Identifies patient using 2 patient identifiers	Fails to identify patient prior to intervening
Prioritizes tasks to ensure most important tasks are completed first	Prioritizes all tasks appropriately, assists others with staying on task when necessary	Prioritizes most tasks appropriately, self-corrects when needed	Fails to prioritize tasks by most urgent needs (fails to place oxygen before notifying MD, for example)
Performs all tasks in an efficient and competent manner	Performs all tasks efficiently and competently, provides coaching to others when necessary	Works efficiently with minimal delays in providing interventions	Fails to work efficiently, makes critical errors that delay providing interventions
Specific Objectives			
Verifies the physician's order	Reviews chart and verifies written physician order	Verifies order verbally with physician or other healthcare provider	Does not verify physician's orders
Assesses the patient	Performs assessment rapidly and correctly, including ALL 8 components as follows: Breath sounds, HR, RR, FiO_2, BP, SpO_2, physical assessment (appearance), and history of illness AND considers other assessment parameters, such as WOB, temperature, and past medical history	Performs assessment rapidly and correctly, obtains 7 of 8 as follows: Breath sounds, HR, RR, FIO_2, BP, SpO_2, physical assessment (appearance), and history of illness	Incorrect techniques utilized in assessment, or assessment not completed, or assessment incomplete (< 7)

Objectives	Pass		Needs Improvement
	Exceeds Standards	Meets Standards	Below Standards
Recognizes signs and symptoms of an acute COPD exacerbation	Identifies or verbalizes patient status an acute exacerbation of COPD and independently provides specific patient data as supportive evidence	Identifies or verbalizes patient status as an acute exacerbation of COPD, and is able to provide supportive evidence once prompted	Fails to identify patient status as COPD exacerbation AND is unable to provide any supportive evidence once prompted
Recommends appropriate initial therapies (Oxygen, BiPAP)	Initiates NPPV therapy with settings appropriate to the pathophysiology within 5 minutes of initial patient encounter	Initiates oxygen therapy within 5 minutes of initial patient encounter, at an appropriate flow rate, device, and FIO_2	Fails to initiate either NPPV or oxygen therapy within 5 minutes OR recommends inappropriate therapy or settings
Assesses the patient's response to therapy and modifies treatment plan as appropriate	Reassess patient, including breath sounds, WOB, vitals, and effectiveness of current therapy. Titrates current BiPAP settings to decrease WOB or initiates BiPAP	Reassesses patient, including effectiveness of current therapy AND most of: breath sounds, WOB, and vitals Recommends or titrates BiPAP settings to decrease WOB, or initiates BiPAP	Either does not reassess patient OR fails to identify and make changes to therapy OR continues with inappropriate therapy for patient status
Notifies physician with key information regarding patient's condition	Succinctly and professionally notifies physician of patient's status, including pertinent clinical data.	Succinctly and professionally notifies physician of patient's status, including pertinent clinical data. Mostly cohesive report to physician.	Fails to provide physician notification OR fails to provide accurate, succinct report

Other Comments for Student:

Evaluator: ______________________________

Student Worksheet

1.1 Jorge Torres

by Janice Dunaway

Student Name:

Personal Reflection

1. Write a SOAP note that summarizes the simulation.

2. List at least 3 things you've learned during this simulation.

3. Body plethysmography on a patient with a history of chronic cough and shortness of breath reveals an increased TLC, FRC, and RV. Spirometry reveals an FEV1 which is 70% of predicted and the FEV1/FVC is 65% of predicted. There is also a decrease in DLCO values. Which of the following diagnosis is MOST consistent with these values?

   A. Pneumonia
   B. Sarcoidosis
   C. Interstitial Lung Disease
   D. COPD

4. A patient with an acute exacerbation of COPD and is admitted through the ED. This patient is known to be a chronic CO_2 retainer. The patient is placed on oxygen via a nasal cannula at 2 L/min. A pulse oximeter reading shows saturation at 86%, and the patient is breathing about 36 breaths/min. Which of the following is the most appropriate initial action of the Respiratory Care Practitioner?

   A. Change device to a nonrebreather mask
   B. Increase the oxygen flow to 6 L/min
   C. Change device to a venturi mask to maintain Pulse oximetry 88-92%
   D. Administer an inhaled corticosteroid

5. A patient admitted with an exacerbation of COPD is placed on BiPAP of 8/4 cm H_2O initially. An ABG is drawn about 30 minutes later, with the following results: pH 7.34, $PaCO_2$ 58 mm Hg, PaO_2 50 torr, HCO_3 28 mEq/L. Which of the following settings is the most appropriate change for this patient?

   A. Increase the IPAP to 10 cm H_2O
   B. Decrease the IPAP to 6 cm H_2O
   C. Increase the EPAP to 6 cm H_2O
   D. Both A and C

Further Reflection

6. At what point should a patient in acute exacerbation of COPD be considered for admission to the hospital? What signs and symptoms should be present?

7. According to the Global Initiative for Chronic Obstructive Lung Disease (GOLD), what are the classifications or stages of COPD?

PERFORMANCE CHECKLIST

Student Name: ____________________ Date Performed: ____________________

Objectives	Pass		Needs Improvement
	Exceeds Standards	Meets Standards	Below Standards
General Objectives			
Performs hand hygiene at all appropriate intervention points	Intervenes and reminds others of need for PPE and hand hygiene	Washes hands prior to all contact points, including in between interventions	Fails to perform hand hygiene prior to patient contact or at any other intervention point
Introduces self to the patient and/or family professionally	Introduces self to patient and family, displays friendly, professional behavior at all times	Introduces self to patient and family in a professional manner	Fails to introduce self to patient and/or family, OR fails to introduce self professionally
Identifies the patient using a minimum of 2 patient identifiers	Identifies patient using 2 identifiers and explains reasoning to patient briefly	Identifies patient using 2 patient identifiers	Fails to identify patient prior to intervening
Prioritizes tasks to ensure most important tasks are completed first	Prioritizes all tasks appropriately, assists others with staying on task when necessary	Prioritizes most tasks appropriately, self-corrects when needed	Fails to prioritize tasks by most urgent needs (fails to place oxygen before notifying MD, for example)
Performs all tasks in an efficient and competent manner	Performs all tasks efficiently and competently, provides coaching to others when necessary	Works efficiently with minimal delays in providing interventions	Fails to work efficiently, makes critical errors that delay providing interventions
Specific Objectives			
Patient assessment and initial therapeutic intervention	Meets Standards, AND: Recognizes all 5 abnormal vitals signs AND initiates BOTH O2 therapy and SABA by SVN.	Performs initial assessment AND recognizes 3 of 5 abnormal vital signs AND initiates oxygen therapy with a min 2 L/min nasal cannula within 7 minutes OR initiates nebulizer therapy with a bronchodilator within 7 minutes.	Fails to meet one or more of the standards

Objectives	Pass		Needs Improvement
	Exceeds Standards	Meets Standards	Below Standards
Re-assessment and re-evaluation	Meets Standards AND Recommends initiation of Heliox therapy	Performs post-treatment assessment AND notifies physician of continued patient distress AND recommends repetitive or continuous bronchodilator therapy AND increases oxygen to a minimum 4 L/min nasal cannula	Fails to meet one or more standards
Recommendation, Implementation, and Documentation	Recommends continued bronchodilator therapy and/or heliox therapy AND implements recommended intervention(s) AND documents interventions and pt status	Implements recommended intervention AND documents interventions and pt status	Requests further orders from physician AND documents interventions and pt status

Other Comments for Student:

Evaluator: ______________________________

Student Worksheet

by Janice Dunaway

Student Name:

Personal Reflection

1. Write a SOAP note that summarizes the simulation.

2. List at least 3 things you've learned during this simulation.

NBRC Preparation

3. A student athlete states she gets short of breath while playing soccer, sometimes to the point where she needs to stop playing. Which of the following is the BEST choice for this patient?

   A. Short-acting Beta Agonist 20-30 minutes prior to exercise
   B. Prophylactic antibiotic administration
   C. Mast-Cell Stabilizer
   D. Short-acting Beta Agonist every 4 hours, while awake

4. Which of the following spirometry values is the most useful in quickly categorizing the severity of an asthma exacerbation, the response to treatment, and in predicting the need for hospitalization in adults?
   A. FVC
   B. FEF 25-75%
   C. PEFR
   D. FEV1

Further Reflection

5. According to the National Asthma Education and Prevention Program (NAEPP) Guidelines, what are the classifications of Asthma?

6. A patient with severe airflow obstruction is currently on Oxygen running at 10 L/min via a Nonrebreather. The RCP requests a trial of an 80/20 Heliox mix.

   a. Calculate the actual flow delivered to the patient, assuming a continued need for 10 L/min.

   b. An H cylinder is delivered, with 2,200 PSIG reading on the gauge. Assuming you change the cylinder out at 500 PSIG, how long will this cylinder last running at 10 L/min?

PERFORMANCE CHECKLIST

Student Name: ____________________ Date Performed: ____________________

Learner Objectives	Pass		Needs Improvement
	Exceeds Standards	Meets Standards	Below Standards
General Objectives			
Performs hand hygiene at all appropriate intervention points	Intervenes and reminds others of need for PPE and hand hygiene	Washes hands prior to all contact points, including in between interventions	Fails to perform hand hygiene prior to patient contact or at any other intervention point
Introduces self to the patient and/or family professionally	Introduces self to patient and family, displays friendly, professional behavior at all times	Introduces self to patient and family in a professional manner	Fails to introduce self to patient and/or family, OR fails to introduce self professionally
Identifies the patient using a minimum of 2 patient identifiers	Identifies patient using 2 identifiers and explains reasoning to patient briefly	Identifies patient using 2 patient identifiers	Fails to identify patient prior to intervening
Prioritizes tasks to ensure most important tasks are completed first	Prioritizes all tasks appropriately, assists others with staying on task when necessary	Prioritizes most tasks appropriately, self-corrects when needed	Fails to prioritize tasks by most urgent needs (fails to place oxygen before notifying MD, for example)
Performs all tasks in an efficient and competent manner	Performs all tasks efficiently and competently, provides coaching to others when necessary	Works efficiently with minimal delays in providing interventions	Fails to work efficiently, makes critical errors that delay providing interventions
Specific Objectives			
Student performs initial patient assessment and recognizes abnormal vital signs (SpO2, HR)	Meets standards AND Recognizes high pressure alarm AND notifies physician of alarm	Correctly analyzes admission ABG AND performs full assessment AND performs full ventilator check AND notices alarm but does not attempt to correct	Fails to meet one or more of the standards
Student correctly analyzes ABG values: **A. Acute Respiratory Acidosis with severe Hypoxemia** **B. P/F ratio 32**	Student correctly analyzes ABG and interprets shunting as indicated by P/F ratio	Student correctly analyzes ABG AND Oxygenation status	Student incorrectly analyzes ABG or Oxygenation status, or both

Learner Objectives	Pass		Needs Improvement
	Exceeds Standards	Meets Standards	Below Standards
Correctly interprets CXR and identifies changing ventilator condition	Systematically assesses CXR, possibly looks for additional CXR to compare against current AND utilizes graphics in examination of lung dynamics	Utilizes CXR in assessment, identifies bilaterally infiltrates (ground glass) AND identifies unacceptable measures on ventilator	Fails to utilize CXR during assessment process, OR unable to identify key elements of CXR OR fails to identify unacceptable measures on ventilator
Student obtains further diagnostic testing after notifying physician	Orders CXR and identifies ground glass appearance AND completes repeat ABG and correctly analyzes values AND verbalizes probability of pt with ARDS. Notifies physician of likelihood of ARDS	Completes repeat ABG AND orders CXR Notifies physician for diagnosis	Does not contact physician for further orders
Correctly analyzes follow-up ABG: Acute Respiratory Acidosis with severe Hypoxemia	Correctly analyzes follow-up ABG and specifically calculates A-a gradient, P/F ratio, or other indicator of shunt	Correctly analyzes follow-up ABG	Fails to correctly analyze follow-up ABG
Recognizes need to initiate lung protection, including Vt, RR, and Mode	Makes recommendations as outlined AND demonstrates strong understanding of pathophysiology, including use of optimal PEEP and need for lung protection	Recognizes inappropriate settings and makes recommendations as outlined, minimally recommending lowering Vt and increasing RR	Does not recognize need to initiate lung protective strategy, or leaves in Volume Control but fails to look at PIP and Pplat relationship.
Considers advanced options for correction of ABG results (proning, IRV, APRV, ECMO, iNO, etc.)	Clearly communicates a strategy to address ventilatory needs, with careful considerations of indications, contraindications, and hazards of strategy	Recognizes need to make further changes to ventilatory strategy	Fails to recognize need for changes, OR makes inappropriate recommendations in context of pathophysiology
Notifies physician of patient's ongoing condition, and recommendations or actions	Provides a clear, concise report to physician that includes condition AND recommendations or actions	Provides report to physician, requiring minimal cues to present appropriate information concisely	Fails to notify physician during simulation, or fails to provide a clear and concise report, even with cues

Other Comments for Student:

Evaluator: ______________________________

Student Worksheet

by Sherry Whiteman

Student Name:

Personal Reflection

1. Write a SOAP note that summarizes the simulation.

2. List at least 3 things you've learned during this simulation.

3. Which of the following are factors found to be associated with ARDS?

   I. Oxygen Toxicity
   II. Shock
   III. Thoracic Trauma
   IV. Radiation-induced Lung Injury

   A. I and III only
   B. I and IV only
   C. II, III, and IV only
   D. I, II, III, and IV

4. In severe ARDS, the Chest X-Ray will have what type of appearance?
   A. Translucent
   B. Slightly opaque
   C. Butterfly
   D. Ground-glass

5. A patient with ARDS requires Mechanical Ventilation. What should the tidal volume be initially set at (assuming plateau < 30 cm H_2O) for a female patient that if 5'6" tall and weighs 142 lbs?

   A. 200 mL
   B. 400 mL
   C. 600 mL
   D. 800 mL

6. According to the ARDSnet protocol, what is the oxygenation goal for a patient with ARDS?

   A. 50 -75 mm Hg
   B. 55 - 80 mm Hg
   C. 70 - 95 mm Hg
   D. 80 - 100 mm Hg

7. The Respiratory Care Practitioner may allow the $PaCO_2$ of an ARDS patient to be higher-than-normal, a result of decreased tidal volumes, and increased metabolic rates. The term used to describe this ventilatory strategy is:

   A. Controlled hyperventilation
   B. Permissive hypercapnea
   C. Iatrogenic hyperventilation
   D. Controlled hyperacidosis

Further Reflection

8. What are the 4 specific criteria we use to determine a patient has ARDS?

9. A patient is currently on a 40% Venturi Mask, having a normal minute ventilation, with the following ABG results:

pH	7.35
$PaCO_2$	45 mm Hg
PaO_2	70 torr,
HCO_3^-	25 mEq/L

a. What is the patient's P/F ratio (show your work)?

b. What is the significance of the P/F ratio in general (what does it tell us clinically)?
Bonus: What doesn't it tell us (what does it NOT take into account)?

PERFORMANCE CHECKLIST

Student Name: ______________________ Date Performed: ______________________

Learner Objectives	Pass		Needs Improvement
	Exceeds Standards	Meets Standards	Below Standards
General Objectives			
Performs hand hygiene at all appropriate intervention points	Intervenes and reminds others of need for PPE and hand hygiene	Washes hands prior to all contact points, including in between interventions	Fails to perform hand hygiene prior to patient contact or at any other intervention point
Introduces self to the patient and/or family professionally	Introduces self to patient and family, displays friendly, professional behavior at all times	Introduces self to patient and family in a professional manner	Fails to introduce self to patient and/or family, OR fails to introduce self professionally
Identifies the patient using a minimum of 2 patient identifiers	Identifies patient using 2 identifiers and explains reasoning to patient briefly	Identifies patient using 2 patient identifiers	Fails to identify patient prior to intervening
Prioritizes tasks to ensure most important tasks are completed first	Prioritizes all tasks appropriately, assists others with staying on task when necessary	Prioritizes most tasks appropriately, self-corrects when needed	Fails to prioritize tasks by most urgent needs (fails to place oxygen before notifying MD, for example)
Performs all tasks in an efficient and competent manner	Performs all tasks efficiently and competently, provides coaching to others when necessary	Works efficiently with minimal delays in providing interventions	Fails to work efficiently, makes critical errors that delay providing interventions
Specific Objectives			
Verifies the physician's order		Verifies the physician's order	Fails to verify the physician's order
Assesses the patient	Systematically but concisely assesses the patient, using appropriate verbal and nonverbal language	Assesses patient appropriately, with several steps not systematic, or not appropriately concise	Fails to assess patient, or does not do so in logical/systematic order

Learner Objectives	Pass		Needs Improvement
	Exceeds Standards	Meets Standards	Below Standards
Acts professionally and caring during simulation	Provides comfort measures to the patient AND family. Notifies physician, using effective communication. Offers supportive resources to the family	Provides comfort measures to the patient. Notifies physician of occurrence and uses effective communication	Does NOT provide comfort measures OR notify physician or use effective communication skills during simulation
Communicates professionally with family	Assesses family's understanding of patient's disease state AND discusses treatment options with family	Discusses treatment with family in a caring manner	Does not effectively communicate with family regarding patient disease state or treatment options
Notifies physician of patient's condition	Notifies physician of patient's condition using professional language AND provides very succinct, relevant details	Notifies physician of condition using professional language and covers all key aspects	Fails to notify physician OR neglects to mention important aspects

Other Comments for Student:

Evaluator: ________________________________

Student Worksheet

1.4 Virgil Banks

by Janice Dunaway

Student Name:

Personal Reflection

1. Write a SOAP note that summarizes the simulation.

2. List at least 3 things you've learned during this simulation.

Further Reflection

3. In healthcare, what is autonomy and what conditions must exist for a patient to be declared autonomous?

4. If a patient is considered incompetent (a legal designation) to make healthcare decisions, who has the right to decide for them?

5. What do the terms Beneficence and Non-Maleficence mean?

6. What other supporting resources might be available to offer this family during this time?

PERFORMANCE CHECKLIST

Student Name: ______________________ Date Performed: ______________________

Learner Objectives	Pass		Needs Improvement
	Exceeds Standards	**Meets Standards**	**Below Standards**
General Objectives			
Performs hand hygiene at all appropriate intervention points	Intervenes and reminds others of need for PPE and hand hygiene	Washes hands prior to all contact points, including in between interventions	Fails to perform hand hygiene prior to patient contact or at any other intervention point
Introduces self to the patient and/or family professionally	Introduces self to patient and family, displays friendly, professional behavior at all times	Introduces self to patient and family in a professional manner	Fails to introduce self to patient and/or family, OR fails to introduce self professionally
Identifies the patient using a minimum of 2 patient identifiers	Identifies patient using 2 identifiers and explains reasoning to patient briefly	Identifies patient using 2 patient identifiers	Fails to identify patient prior to intervening
Prioritizes tasks to ensure most important tasks are completed first	Prioritizes all tasks appropriately, assists others with staying on task when necessary	Prioritizes most tasks appropriately, self-corrects when needed	Fails to prioritize tasks by most urgent needs (fails to place oxygen before notifying MD, for example)
Performs all tasks in an efficient and competent manner	Performs all tasks efficiently and competently, provides coaching to others when necessary	Works efficiently with minimal delays in providing interventions	Fails to work efficiently, makes critical errors that delay providing interventions
Specific Objectives			
Performs initial patient assessment and recognizes abnormal vital signs	Obtains HR, RR, Temperature, BS, SpO_2, and patient's stated symptoms (diaphoresis, SOB, increased cough, weakness) AND verbalizes that they are abnormal AND performs a focused patient history AND initiates 2 L/min nasal cannula AND inquires about pt CXR	Obtains 4 of 6 assessment findings [HR, RR, Temp, SpO2, and symptoms (diaphoresis, SOB, cough, weakness)] AND verbalizes that they are abnormal AND initiates 2 L/min nasal cannula	Fails to meet one or more of the standards

Learner Objectives	Pass		Needs Improvement
	Exceeds Standards	Meets Standards	Below Standards
Determines cause of patient state	Meets Standards AND Creates a care plan for patient care that includes problem, intervention, and goal/outcome AND verbalizes possible alternatives to therapy based on patient learning barriers	Correctly interprets CXR as atelectasis AND discusses possible causes of atelectasis AND notifies physician of findings to request orders for treatment	Fails to meet one or more of the Standards
Performs corrective therapy and communicates with patient	Meets Stadards AND Communciates need for intervention with patient AND conduscts patient education appropriate for patient cognition and abilities	Begins to initiate SMI 10 breaths Q1 while awake or PEP therapy Q4-6 AND evaluates the patient's response to interventions OR initiates therapy according to physician order AND documents interventions and patient's status	Fails to meet one or more of the Standards

Other Comments for Student:

Evaluator: ______________________________

Student Worksheet

by Whiteman, Dunaway, Lewis, Pippin

Student Name:

Personal Reflection

1. Write a SOAP note that summarizes the simulation.

2. List at least 3 things you've learned during this simulation.

3. The loss of alveolar volume, generally caused by the complete deflation and reinflation of alveoli, that is both a consequence and a cause of lung injury is termed:
   A. Biotrauma
   B. Volutrauma
   C. Barotrauma
   D. Atelectrauma

4. Which of the following are types of atelectasis?
   I. Resorptive
   II. Lobar
   III. Compression
   IV. Centrilobular

   A. I and III only
   B. II and IV only
   C. I, II, and III only
   D. I, II, III, and IV

5. Lung expansion therapies work to increase lung volumes by increasing which of the following?
   A. Airway closing pressure
   B. Transpulmonary pressure
   C. Transpleural pressure
   D. Transchest pressure

Further Reflection

6. Calculate the volume a patient is achieving on a flow-oriented incentive spirometer if that patient has a measured flow of 300 mL/sec, and is performing a 5-second breath-hold.

7. List at least 5 potential positive outcomes that could be included on a respiratory care plan for a patient with a diagnosis of atelectasis.

8. For the outcomes you just developed in the previous question, write an individual treatment plan for a patient with atelectasis.

9. In your own words, describe how you would instruct a patient on Positive Expiratory Pressure (PEP) therapy.

PERFORMANCE CHECKLIST

Student Name: ______________________ Date Performed: ______________________

Learner Objectives	Pass		Needs Improvement
	Exceeds Standards	Meets Standards	Below Standards
General Objectives			
Performs hand hygiene at all appropriate intervention points	Intervenes and reminds others of need for PPE and hand hygiene	Washes hands prior to all contact points, including in between interventions	Fails to perform hand hygiene prior to patient contact or at any other intervention point
Introduces self to the patient and/or family professionally	Introduces self to patient and family, displays friendly, professional behavior at all times	Introduces self to patient and family in a professional manner	Fails to introduce self to patient and/or family, OR fails to introduce self professionally
Identifies the patient using a minimum of 2 patient identifiers	Identifies patient using 2 identifiers and explains reasoning to patient briefly	Identifies patient using 2 patient identifiers	Fails to identify patient prior to intervening
Prioritizes tasks to ensure most important tasks are completed first	Prioritizes all tasks appropriately, assists others with staying on task when necessary	Prioritizes most tasks appropriately, self-corrects when needed	Fails to prioritize tasks by most urgent needs (fails to place oxygen before notifying MD, for example)
Performs all tasks in an efficient and competent manner	Performs all tasks efficiently and competently, provides coaching to others when necessary	Works efficiently with minimal delays in providing interventions	Fails to work efficiently, makes critical errors that delay providing interventions
Specific Objectives			
Gathers equipment and explains monitoring (capnograph, pulse oximetry)	Meets Standards, AND Verifies location of manual resuscitator and mask AND location of O_2 source	Gathers noninvasive $ETCO_2$ monitor (via NC) and SpO_2, places both on patient and explains to patient adequately using appropriate language AND monitors patient closely	Fails to meet one or more of the Standards

Learner Objectives	Pass		Needs Improvement
	Exceeds Standards	Meets Standards	Below Standards
Recognizes hypoventilation and performs appropriate corrective measures	Meets Standards, and Identifies hypoventilaton within 1 minute AND recommends adminsitration of an opiate antagonist	Monitors patient closely AND identifies hypoventilaton within 2 minutes of beginning of occurrence AND initiates rescue breathing with manual resuscitator/mask and oxygen	Fails to meet one or more of the Standards

Other Comments for Student:

Evaluator: ______________________________

Student Worksheet

by Janice Dunaway

Student Name:

Personal Reflection

1. Write a SOAP note that summarizes the simulation.

2. List at least 3 things you've learned during this simulation.

NBRC Preparation

1. A sudden loss or absence of waveform and $ETCO_2$ reading may be seen in all of the following except?

   A. Esophageal intubation
   B. Airway disconnect from the ventilator
   C. Obstructed endotracheal tube
   D. Bronchospasm

2. A sudden exponential decrease in the $ETCO_2$ may be seen in all of the following except:

   A. Rebreathing CO_2
   B. Massive blood loss
   C. Circulatory failure with continued ventilation
   D. Pulmonary embolism

3. Which of the following BEST describes the following capnogram?

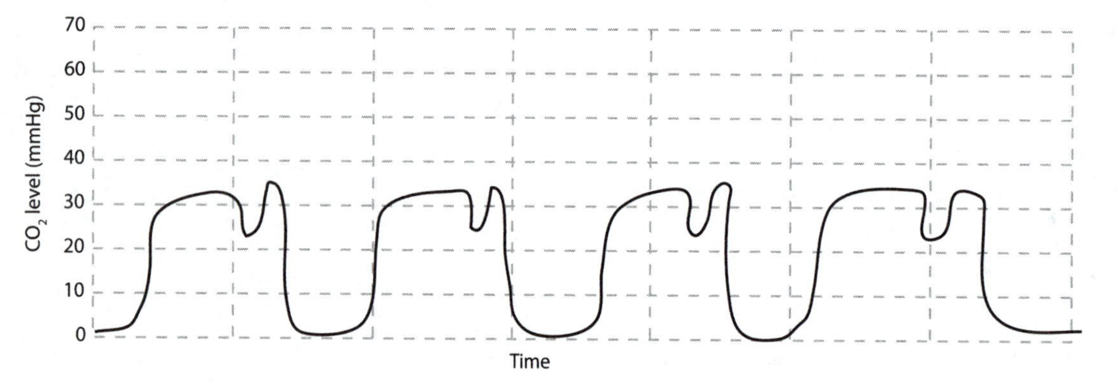

   A. Hypothermia
   B. Sedation
   C. Decreasing cardiac output
   D. Curare cleft

4. A patient on mechanical ventilation has a mainstream capnograph attached to the ventilator circuit to monitor exhaled CO_2 levels following an MVA. The patient has an acute head injury and the physician wants to maintain the CO_2 level at 35 mm hg. The capnograph begins to show a characteristic shark fin appearance. Which of the following conditions is the most common cause of this type of waveform?

   A. Hypoventilation
   B. Hypervolemia
   C. Airflow obstruction
   D. Misplaced endotracheal tube

Further Reflection

5. Describe the three types of capnography and the common uses for each.

6. Describe the relationship between cardiac output and $ETCO_2$.

7. A patient being monitored with capnography has a strong radial pulse and normal blood pressure, but a low $ETCO_2$ and a diminished waveform. What are some probable causes for this scenario?

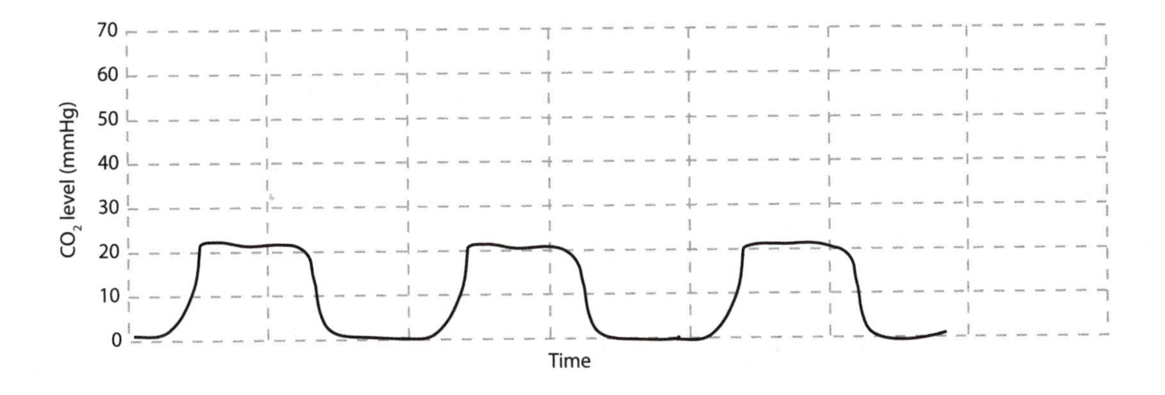

8. A patient on mechanical ventilation is also being monitored with capnography. The following capnography waveform shows an increasing elevated baseline but stable $ETCO_2$ reading. What may be some probable causes for this kind of waveform?

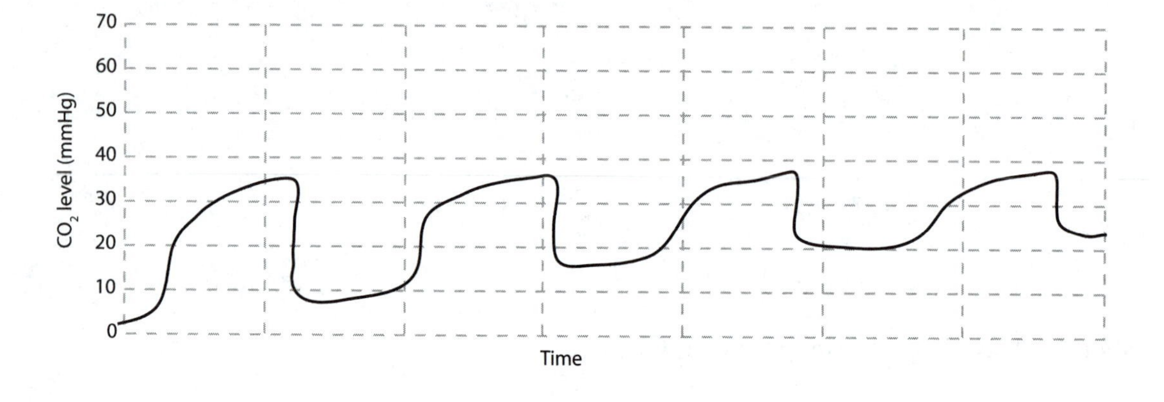

PERFORMANCE CHECKLIST

Student Name: ____________________ Date Performed: ____________________

Learner Objectives	Pass		Needs Improvement
	Exceeds Standards	Meets Standards	Below Standards
General Objectives			
Performs hand hygiene at all appropriate intervention points	Intervenes and reminds others of need for PPE and hand hygiene	Washes hands prior to all contact points, including in between interventions	Fails to perform hand hygiene prior to patient contact or at any other intervention point
Introduces self to the patient and/or family professionally	Introduces self to patient and family, displays friendly, professional behavior at all times	Introduces self to patient and family in a professional manner	Fails to introduce self to patient and/or family, OR fails to introduce self professionally
Identifies the patient using a minimum of 2 patient identifiers	Identifies patient using 2 identifiers and explains reasoning to patient briefly	Identifies patient using 2 patient identifiers	Fails to identify patient prior to intervening
Prioritizes tasks to ensure most important tasks are completed first	Prioritizes all tasks appropriately, assists others with staying on task when necessary	Prioritizes most tasks appropriately, self-corrects when needed	Fails to prioritize tasks by most urgent needs (fails to place oxygen before notifying MD, for example)
Performs all tasks in an efficient and competent manner	Performs all tasks efficiently and competently, provides coaching to others when necessary	Works efficiently with minimal delays in providing interventions	Fails to work efficiently, makes critical errors that delay providing interventions
Specific Objectives			
Performs complete patient assessment and recognizes abnormal vital signs	Meets Standards, AND Identifies 5 or more of the 6 patient symptoms AND verbalizes possible cause of distress as CHF	Performs thorough, systematic patient assessment AND identifies 4 of 6 patient symptoms: hypoxemia, hypertensive state, tachycardia, bi-basilar crackles, peripheral edema, and SOB AND requests CXR and ABG AND titrates O_2 appropriately AND notifies MD of findings	Fails to meet one or more of the Standards

Learner Objectives	Pass		Needs Improvement
	Exceeds Standards	Meets Standards	Below Standards
Recommends and initiates appropriate treatment, notifying family **A. Oxygen therapy** **B. Non-invasive Ventilation** **C. Pharmacologics (diueretics)**	Meets Standards, AND Places patient on adequate CPAP or BiPAP with adequate O_2 (40% or greater recommded) AND verbalizes need for pharmacologic intervention such as loop diuretics	Identifies cause of distress as CHF AND titrates O_2 up appropriately AND communicates patient status to family, adhering to HIPAA guidelines	Fails to meet one or more of the Standards
Modifies therapy according to diagnostic test results	Meets Standards, AND Obtains or requests ABG	Requests follow-up ABG from MD AND correctly interprets ABG results (complete interpretation of Acute Respiratory Acidosis, including oxygenation) AND either now places pt on CPAP or BiPAP with adequate settings, or titrates settings appropriately AND evaluates patient's response to interventions	Fails to meet one or more of the Standards

Other Comments for Student:

Evaluator: ______________________________

Student Worksheet

1.7 Helen Edwards

by Janice Dunaway

Student Name:

Personal Reflection

1. Write a SOAP note that summarizes the simulation.

2. List at least 3 things you've learned during this simulation.

3. A patient on CPAP of 5 cm H_2O and an F_IO_2 0.60 (60%). The following ABG result was drawn 30 minutes after the patient was placed on the CPAP:

pH	7.43
$PaCO_2$	43 mm Hg
HCO_3	22 mEq/L
PaO_2	64 mm Hg

Which of the following represents the next best action by the RCP?

A. Decrease the EPAP level
B. Increase the EPAP level
C. Increase the Oxygen % to 70%
D. Intubate the patient and place on volume ventilation

4. A patient presents to the emergency room with a diagnosis of congestive heart failure. The patient's EKG shows tall, spiked "T" waves. Which of the following statements best reflects the reason for this finding?

A. Excessive work of breathing
B. Accumulation of sodium from fluid retention
C. Accumulation of potassium from diuretic use
D. Respiratory alkalosis

5. Which of the following best depicts a typical CXR on a patient diagnosed with congestive heart failure?

I. Consolidation
II. Perihilar infiltrates
III. Kerley B Lines
IV. Air Bronchogram

A. I and IV
B. II and III
C. I and III
D. II and IV

Further Reflection

6. What are the signs and symptoms of congestive heart failure?

7. Describe the differences between cardiogenic pulmonary edema (hydrostatic) and non-cardiogenic pulmonary edema (non-hydrostatic) with an emphasis on hydrostatic and osmotic pressures.

   How do the treatments vary between cardiogenic and non-cardiogenic pulmonary edema?

PERFORMANCE CHECKLIST

Student Name: ______________________ Date Performed: ______________________

Learner Objectives	Pass		Needs Improvement
	Exceeds Standards	Meets Standards	Below Standards
General Objectives			
Performs hand hygiene at all appropriate intervention points	Intervenes and reminds others of need for PPE and hand hygiene	Washes hands prior to all contact points, including in between interventions	Fails to perform hand hygiene prior to patient contact or at any other intervention point
Introduces self to the patient and/or family professionally	Introduces self to patient and family, displays friendly, professional behavior at all times	Introduces self to patient and family in a professional manner	Fails to introduce self to patient and/or family, OR fails to introduce self professionally
Identifies the patient using a minimum of 2 patient identifiers	Identifies patient using 2 identifiers and explains reasoning to patient briefly	Identifies patient using 2 patient identifiers	Fails to identify patient prior to intervening
Prioritizes tasks to ensure most important tasks are completed first	Prioritizes all tasks appropriately, assists others with staying on task when necessary	Prioritizes most tasks appropriately, self-corrects when needed	Fails to prioritize tasks by most urgent needs (fails to place oxygen before notifying MD, for example)
Performs all tasks in an efficient and competent manner	Performs all tasks efficiently and competently, provides coaching to others when necessary	Works efficiently with minimal delays in providing interventions	Fails to work efficiently, makes critical errors that delay providing interventions
Specific Objectives			
Performs initial patient assessment	Meets Standards AND Assesses patient systematically and concisely AND identifies bradypnea and diminished LOC within 1 minute AND considers the use of an NPA/OPA adjunct	Performs patient assessment AND identifies bradypnea and diminished LOC within 2 minutes of entering room AND initiates rescue breathing	Fails to meet one or more of the Standards

Learner Objectives	Pass		Needs Improvement
	Exceeds Standards	**Meets Standards**	**Below Standards**
Determines cause of diminished LOC, orders and interprets: **A. Toxicology screen** **B. ABG** **C. Electrolyte panel** **D. EKG and/or Heart monitor**	Meets Standards, AND Immediately requests all 6 tests/procedures	Obtains history of present illness (HPI) from roommate and/or paramedics AND requests Chem Panel and EKG and 2 of 3: ABG, 12-lead, CXR, and toxicology screen	Fails to meet one or more of the Standards
Correctly determines cause of diminished LOC and initiates supportive/corrective therapies	Meets Standards, AND Prepares efficiently for intubation AND correctly performs intubation procedure	Identifies electrolyte imbalance as cause of patient status AND recommends intubation and mechanical ventilation	Fails to meet one or more of the Standards

Other Comments for Student:

Evaluator: ______________________________

Student Worksheet

by Janice Dunaway

Student Name:

Personal Reflection

1. Write a SOAP note that summarizes the simulation.

2. List at least 3 things you've learned during this simulation.

1. Which of the following patients would to be at the greatest risk for developing hypernatremia?

   A. 50 year old with pneumonia, fever, and diaphoresis
   B. 60 year old with congestive heart failure
   C. 40 year old with nausea, vomiting, and diarrhea
   D. 70 year old with dehydration and a Community Acquired Pneumonia (CAP)

2. A patient is experiencing muscle cramps, numbness, and tingling of the extremities, and twitching of the facial muscle and eyelid. This assessment is consistent with which of the following?

   A. Hypokalemia
   B. Hypernatremia
   C. Hypermagnesemia
   D. Hypocalcemia

3. The electrolyte results of an assigned patient notes that the potassium level is 5.4 mEq/L. Which of the following would be expected on the electrocardiogram as a result of this laboratory value?

   A. ST depression
   B. Inverted T wave
   C. Prominent U wave
   D. Tall peaked T waves

Further Reflection

4. Discuss the actions of the sodium- potassium pump and some of the complications that happen with an imbalance.

4. In your own words, describe how positive pressure ventilation may affect a patient's fluid balance.

6. Fill out the chart on the following page.

Electrolyte	Normal Range	Clinical Significance	Term associated with A) Increased level B) Decreased level	List 1 cause for each abnormal condition
Sodium				
Chloride				
Potassium				
Calcium				
Magnesium				
Phosphate				

PERFORMANCE CHECKLIST

Student Name: ____________________ Date Performed: ____________________

Learner Objectives	Pass		Needs Improvement
	Exceeds Standards	Meets Standards	Below Standards
General Objectives			
Performs hand hygiene at all appropriate intervention points	Intervenes and reminds others of need for PPE and hand hygiene	Washes hands prior to all contact points, including in between interventions	Fails to perform hand hygiene prior to patient contact or at any other intervention point
Introduces self to the patient and/or family professionally	Introduces self to patient and family, displays friendly, professional behavior at all times	Introduces self to patient and family in a professional manner	Fails to introduce self to patient and/or family, OR fails to introduce self professionally
Identifies the patient using a minimum of 2 patient identifiers	Identifies patient using 2 identifiers and explains reasoning to patient briefly	Identifies patient using 2 patient identifiers	Fails to identify patient prior to intervening
Prioritizes tasks to ensure most important tasks are completed first	Prioritizes all tasks appropriately, assists others with staying on task when necessary	Prioritizes most tasks appropriately, self-corrects when needed	Fails to prioritize tasks by most urgent needs (fails to place oxygen before notifying MD, for example)
Performs all tasks in an efficient and competent manner	Performs all tasks efficiently and competently, provides coaching to others when necessary	Works efficiently with minimal delays in providing interventions	Fails to work efficiently, makes critical errors that delay providing interventions
Specific Objectives			
Performs initial patient assessment and recognizes abnormal findings **A. Hypoxemia (SpO_2)** **B. Paradoxical chest wall** **C. Hypotensive (BP)** **D. Tachypnea (RR)**	Meets Standards, AND Idnetifies all signs and symptoms	Performs thorough, systematic patient assessment AND Identifies a minimum of 3: Hypoxemia, Paradoxical chest wall movement, diminished LOC, hypotension, tachypnea AND requests CXR and ABG	Fails to meet one or more of the Standards

Learner Objectives	Pass		Needs Improvement
	Exceeds Standards	Meets Standards	Below Standards
Identifies cause of distress and makes appropriate therapeutic recommendations, including intubation and mechanical ventilation	Meets Standards, AND Correctly identifies distress with flail chest as most likely cause AND recommends appropriate ventilator settings	Correctly identifies patient as being in distress, but does not identify flail chest, AND correctly interprets ABG (including oxygenation) AND recommends intubation and mechanical ventilation	Fails to meet one or more of the Standards
Initiates therapeutic interventions with recommended settings: **• P-A/C or V-A/C (or other appropriate support mode)** **• Vt 5-8 mL/kg** **• PEEP +5 cmH_2O** **• *f* 10-15/min** **• FIO_2 1.0**	Meets Standards, AND Verifies appropriateness of initial settings by observing patient, return ventilator values, and loops/scalars	Intubates patient AND initiates mechanical ventilation with appropriate settings AND records initial settings	Fails to meet one or more of the Standards
Continues to monitor patient and make modifications to settings as clinically appropriate	Meets Standards AND Does not require prompting for ABG AND makes recommendations for appropriate changes (typically decreases FIO_2, Increases RR, Doesn't alter Vt if in range, etc.)	Obtains ABG within 30 simulated minutes after intubation OR requires prompting for ABG AND makes basic recommendations for appropriate changes but may not be optimal (but does not cause harm) AND monitors patient's response AND notifies MD of changes AND documents interventions	Fails to meet one or more of the Standards

Other Comments for Student:

Evaluator: ______________________________

Student Worksheet

by Sherry Whiteman

Student Name:

Personal Reflection

1. Write a SOAP note that summarizes the simulation.

2. List at least 3 things you've learned during this simulation.

NBRC Preparation

1. Mechanical ventilation is usually needed for ______ days to allow a flail chest to heal.

   A. 1 - 2
   B. 10 - 15
   C. 5 - 10
   D. 2 - 3

2. Shunting of air from one lung to another is called ________________.

   A. Painting
   B. Shunting
   C. Bidirectional flow
   D. Pendelluft

3. How does the chest wall move in the area directly beneath the flail chest during inspiration?

   A. Sink inward
   B. Bulge outward
   C. Does not move
   D. Lags behind typical movement

4. Lung compression and atelectasis that results from pendelluft will cause which of the following?

   I. Venous admixture
   II. Decreased V/Q ratio
   III. Increased V/Q ratio
   IV. Increased P_AO_2

   A. I only
   B. II and III only
   C. I and II only
   D. I, II, III, and IV

Further Reflection

1. Many hemodynamic indices are altered in a patient experiencing severe flail chest. For the following indices, indicate the normal value, how the value is altered and identify one noninvasive method for correcting this alteration.

	CVP	PAP	CO	LVSWI	SVR
Normal Range					
Increase or Decrease with Flail Chest?					
Clinical Strategy to fix					

2. Patients with flail chest often develop hypoxemia. Explain why and identify two therapies that would alleviate the hypoxemia, describing how each would work to treat the hypoxemia.

PERFORMANCE CHECKLIST

Student Name: ______________________ Date Performed: ______________________

Learner Objectives	Pass		Needs Improvement
	Exceeds Standards	Meets Standards	Below Standards
General Objectives			
Performs hand hygiene at all appropriate intervention points	Intervenes and reminds others of need for PPE and hand hygiene	Washes hands prior to all contact points, including in between interventions	Fails to perform hand hygiene prior to patient contact or at any other intervention point
Introduces self to the patient and/ or family professionally	Introduces self to patient and family, displays friendly, professional behavior at all times	Introduces self to patient and family in a professional manner	Fails to introduce self to patient and/ or family, OR fails to introduce self professionally
Identifies the patient using a minimum of 2 patient identifiers	Identifies patient using 2 identifiers and explains reasoning to patient briefly	Identifies patient using 2 patient identifiers	Fails to identify patient prior to intervening
Prioritizes tasks to ensure most important tasks are completed first	Prioritizes all tasks appropriately, assists others with staying on task when necessary	Prioritizes most tasks appropriately, self-corrects when needed	Fails to prioritize tasks by most urgent needs (fails to place oxygen before notifying MD, for example)
Performs all tasks in an efficient and competent manner	Performs all tasks efficiently and competently, provides coaching to others when necessary	Works efficiently with minimal delays in providing interventions	Fails to work efficiently, makes critical errors that delay providing interventions
Specific Objectives			
Performs initial patient assessment and recognizes abnormal vital signs; performs a focused patient history	Performs concise systematic assessment, identifies signs and symptoms of respiratory distress, and obtains full patient history. Shows thoroughness in assessment	Identifies signs and symptoms as a result of assessment; obtains patient history	Fails to perform initial patient assessment OR fails to recognize abnormal vitals signs OR does not use systematic approach which results in potential delay of action

Learner Objectives	Pass		Needs Improvement
	Exceeds Standards	Meets Standards	Below Standards
Presents appropriate therapeutic and monitoring recommendations to MD: **A. Oxygen therapy** **B. Vital capacity (q 4-6 hrs)** **C. Negative Inspiratory Force (q 4-16 hrs)** **D. Peak flow (q 4-6 hrs)**	Meets Standards, AND Also recommends Peak Flow and independently explains purpose of each: VC, NIF, Peak Flow	Initiates O_2 therapy with around 2 L/min NC AND recommends VC and NIF.	Fails to meet one or more of the Standards
Identifies potential cause of illness as Gullain-Barre Syndrome	Differentiates between Myasthenia Gravis and Gullain-Barre Syndrome, correctly identifies by symptoms as GBS, is able to discuss intelligently as needed	Identifies neurological disorder, identifies as either Myasthenia Gravis or Guillain-Barre Syndrome and works to identify	Fails to identify as a neurological disorders, makes no mention of Guillain-Barre Syndrome or Myasthenia Gravis
Correctly performs and interprets Vital Capacity, Negative Inspiratory Force, and Peak flow in spontaneously breathing patient	Performs technique of all 3 tests competently, Calculates all actual values correctly and fully interprets results including critical values. Provides clear instruction to patient on reason for each test and detailed instructions on how to perform effectively. Performs 3 attempts for each, and appropriately identifies highest value with good technique as reported value	Performs technique of Vital Capacity and Negative Inspiratory Force appropriately, and correctly interprets all results. Provides at least basic instruction to the patient regarding reason and technique.	Fails to perform VC OR NIF using correct technique OR fails to recognize critical values in interpretation OR fails to provide basic instruction to patient
Verbalizes when to initiate advanced respiratory support	Identifies critical values AND independently identifies need to act, and provides a plan for further respiratory support	Identifies critical values AND identifies need to act, but does not provide clear plan for further respiratory support	Fails to identify critical values OR fails to identify need to act
Evaluates patient's response to interventions	Independently monitors patient's response and provides clear communication to other team members regarding status	Monitors patient's response appropriately	Fails to monitor patient's response
Notifies physician of patient's condition and documents interventions	Meets Standards, AND Physician notification is very concise	Notifies physician of events leading up to intervention, makes appropriate recommendations, and documents all interventions	Fails to meet one or more of the Standards

Other Comments for Student:

Student Worksheet

by Whiteman, Lewis, Dunaway, Pippin

Student Name:

Personal Reflection

1. Write a SOAP note that summarizes the simulation.

2. List at least 3 things you've learned during this simulation.

3. If diagnosed early, patients with Guillain-Barré Syndrome have a(n) ______________ prognosis.

   A. Poor
   B. Questionable
   C. Excellent
   D. Unknown

4. The nerve cells of a patient with Guillain-Barré Syndrome will often show which of the following?

I. Demyelation
II. Edema
III. Inflammation
IV. Myelination

   A. I and III
   B. III and IV
   C. I, II, and III
   D. II, III, and IV

5. The onset of Guillain-Barré Syndrome often occurs about how long after a febrile episode?

   A. 1-4 weeks
   B. 6-8 weeks
   C. 10-12 weeks
   D. 3-6 months

6. Of the following, which would you most expect to find in a patient with Guillain-Barré Syndrome?

   I. Paresthesias
   II. Abnormal EMG
   III. Abnormally high Protein level in CSF
   IV. Abnormally low protein level in CSF

   A. I and II only
   B. II and IV only
   C. I, II, and III
   D. I, II, and IV

Further Reflection

1. Patients with Guillain-Barré Syndrome are sometimes said to meet the ***20-30-40*** criteria.
   a. What criteria is being measured?

   b. What is this criteria used to determine?

   c. What action(s) should be considered if the patient meets these criteria?

2. Create a table that compares Guillain-Barré Syndrome with Myasthenia Gravis and Amyotrophic Lateral Sclerosis. In your chart, include a) the nature of the paralysis; b) common causes; b) pertinent lab values (including ABGs); c) treatments; and d) reversibility.

PERFORMANCE CHECKLIST

Student Name: ______________________ Date Performed: ______________________

Learner Objectives	Pass		Needs Improvement
	Exceeds Standards	**Meets Standards**	**Below Standards**
General Objectives			
Performs hand hygiene at all appropriate intervention points	Intervenes and reminds others of need for PPE and hand hygiene	Washes hands prior to all contact points, including in between interventions	Fails to perform hand hygiene prior to patient contact or at any other intervention point
Introduces self to the patient and/or family professionally	Introduces self to patient and family, displays friendly, professional behavior at all times	Introduces self to patient and family in a professional manner	Fails to introduce self to patient and/or family, OR fails to introduce self professionally
Identifies the patient using a minimum of 2 patient identifiers	Identifies patient using 2 identifiers and explains reasoning to patient briefly	Identifies patient using 2 patient identifiers	Fails to identify patient prior to intervening
Prioritizes tasks to ensure most important tasks are completed first	Prioritizes all tasks appropriately, assists others with staying on task when necessary	Prioritizes most tasks appropriately, self-corrects when needed	Fails to prioritize tasks by most urgent needs (fails to place oxygen before notifying MD, for example)
Performs all tasks in an efficient and competent manner	Performs all tasks efficiently and competently, provides coaching to others when necessary	Works efficiently with minimal delays in providing interventions	Fails to work efficiently, makes critical errors that delay providing interventions
Specific Objectives			
Performs initial patient assessment	Meets Standards, AND Reviews CXR findings AND recommends either decreasing set Vt or to a Pressure (or combined) mode of ventilation or optimal PEEP maneuver	Performs systematic initial assessment AND completes ventilator monitoring AND recognizes abnormal hemodynamic values AND notifies MD of findings. May make general recommendations to MD.	Fails to meet one or more of the Standards

Learner Objectives	Pass		Needs Improvement
	Exceeds Standards	Meets Standards	Below Standards
Evaluates patient response to therapeutic interventions	Meets Standards, AND Titrates therapeutic intervention to optimize patient status	Monitors patient response to chosen therapeutic intervention AND notifies MD/RN of patient condition AND documents interventions and patient status	Fails to meet one or more of the Standards

Other Comments for Student:

Evaluator: ______________________________

Student Worksheet

by Janice Dunaway

Student Name:

Personal Reflection

1. Write a SOAP note that summarizes the simulation.

2. List at least 3 things you've learned during this simulation.

3. A patient is being monitored in the ICU with pulmonary artery catheter. The physician asks you for a pulmonary capillary wedge pressure and you inflate the balloon with 1 mL of air. The monitor shows the following waveform. You note the following waveform:

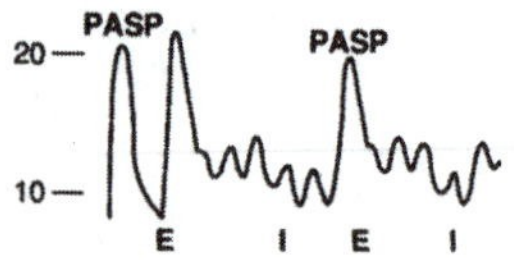

Which of the following is the best choice?

A. The PA catheter has become infected and needs to be removed immediately
B. The Respiratory Therapist needs to inflate the balloon with 1.5 mL of air
C. The Respiratory Therapist needs to withdraw the catheter approximately 2 cm
D. The Respiratory Therapist needs to verify the balloon has 25-30 mm Hg using a cuff manometer.

4. Which of the following conditions could increase the pulmonary vascular resistance and the right ventricular afterload without causing an increase in the pulmonary capillary wedge pressure?

A. Sepsis
B. Peripheral vasodilation
C. Systemic hypertension
D. Chronic Obstructive Pulmonary Disease (COPD)

5. A patient in the medical ICU has the following information collected from the pulmonary artery catheter:

PAP	48/32 mm Hg
PCWP	22 mm Hg
CVP	15 mm Hg
CO	9.0 L

A. Hypovolemia
B. Hypervolemia
C. Acute pulmonary embolus
D. Left ventricular failure

6. Lung compression and atelectasis that results from pendelluft will cause which of the following?

    I. Venous admixture
    II. Decreased V/Q ratio
    III. Increased V/Q ratio
    IV. Increased P_AO_2

    A. I only
    B. II and III only
    C. I and II only
    D. I, II, III, and IV

Further Reflection

7. List 5 causes for a "dampened" waveform when measuring pulmonary artery pressures.

8. During what phase of the breathing cycle should you take a pulmonary capillary wedge pressure? Why?

9. When measuring the pulmonary artery pressure of a patient on mechanical ventilation and PEEP, should the measurements be taken on the ventilator, or should the patient be removed from the ventilator prior to measuring? Why?

10. Describe the importance of proper placement of the transducer when measuring pulmonary artery pressure and cardiac output.

PERFORMANCE CHECKLIST

Student Name: ____________________ Date Performed: ____________________

Learner Objectives	Pass		Needs Improvement
	Exceeds Standards	**Meets Standards**	**Below Standards**
General Objectives			
Performs hand hygiene at all appropriate intervention points	Intervenes and reminds others of need for PPE and hand hygiene	Washes hands prior to all contact points, including in between interventions	Fails to perform hand hygiene prior to patient contact or at any other intervention point
Introduces self to the patient and/or family professionally	Introduces self to patient and family, displays friendly, professional behavior at all times	Introduces self to patient and family in a professional manner	Fails to introduce self to patient and/or family, OR fails to introduce self professionally
Identifies the patient using a minimum of 2 patient identifiers	Identifies patient using 2 identifiers and explains reasoning to patient briefly	Identifies patient using 2 patient identifiers	Fails to identify patient prior to intervening
Prioritizes tasks to ensure most important tasks are completed first	Prioritizes all tasks appropriately, assists others with staying on task when necessary	Prioritizes most tasks appropriately, self-corrects when needed	Fails to prioritize tasks by most urgent needs (fails to place oxygen before notifying MD, for example)
Performs all tasks in an efficient and competent manner	Performs all tasks efficiently and competently, provides coaching to others when necessary	Works efficiently with minimal delays in providing interventions	Fails to work efficiently, makes critical errors that delay providing interventions
Specific Objectives			
Performs rapid initial assessment and initiates immediate interventions	Meets Standards AND Obtains all 8 findings	Obtains 6 out of 8 patient assessment findings AND verbalizes abnormal findings AND initiates O_2 therapy	Fails to meet one or more of the Standards
Identifies increasing distress and performs appropriate diagnostic testing	Meets Standards, AND Communicates effectively with the patient and family members	Identifies increased HR, RR, BP, and pain AND determines need to obtain EKG AND correctly performs EKG AND identifies ST elevation with or without prompting by MD on rhythm strip AND notifies MD of findings	Fails to meet one or more of the Standards

Learner Objectives	Pass		Needs Improvement
	Exceeds Standards	**Meets Standards**	**Below Standards**
Prioritizes care and administers appropriate therapeutic interventions	Initiates O_2 via NRB within 7 minutes of simulation start AND requests Morphine administration AND requests sublingual Nitroglycerin AND requests ASA administration AND identifies STEMI on EKG AND verbalizes considerations for advanced care of patient	Initiates O_2 via NRB within 7 minutes of simulation start AND requests further orders from MD to treat patient pain and discomfort AND identifies irregularity on EKG strip, but may not identify as STEMI	Fails to administer O_2 within 7 minutes OR does not prioritize care of patient with STEMI
Notifies physician of patient's condition	Notifies physician of patient's condition using professional language AND provides very succinct, relevant details	Notifies physician of condition using professional language and covers all key aspects	Fails to notify physician OR neglects to mention important aspects

Other Comments for Student:

Evaluator: ______________________________

Student Worksheet

1.12 Oscar Hensley

by Glenda Pippin

Student Name:

Personal Reflection

1. Write a SOAP note that summarizes the simulation.

2. List at least 3 things you've learned during this simulation.

3. Which of the following conditions are likely to cause chest pain?

   I. Aortic dissection
   II. Pericarditis/Myocarditis
   III. Pulmonary embolus

   A. I only
   B. I and III only
   C. II and III only
   D. I, II, and III

4. Which of the following are indicated for a hypoxic patient with ischemic-type chest pain?

   I. Supplemental oxygen
   II. 12-lead EKG
   III. IV access
   IV. Cardiac bypass surgery
   V. Stress test

   A. I and II only
   B. IV and V only
   C. I, II, and III only
   D. I, II, and IV only

5. Which of the following pharmacologic categories are indicated for ischemic chest pain?

   A. Anticoagulants
   B. Beta-blockers
   C. Calcium channel blockers
   D. All of the above

Further Reflection

6. Which portion of the EKG is assessed to determine if a patient is experiencing an acute myocardial infarction? What is occurring at the cellular level to produce the changes seen on the EKG?

7. If a patient having a Myocardial Infarction remains untreated for an extended period of time, further changes on the EKG may be seen. What changes are seen, and what is indicated by his change?

8. What diagnostic tests or procedures should be performed on a patient with suspected myocardial infarction?

9. List the treatment options for a patient diagnosed with an acute Myocardial Infarction.

PERFORMANCE CHECKLIST

Student Name: ______________________ Date Performed: ______________________

Learner Objectives	Pass		Needs Improvement
	Exceeds Standards	Meets Standards	Below Standards
General Objectives			
Performs hand hygiene at all appropriate intervention points	Intervenes and reminds others of need for PPE and hand hygiene	Washes hands prior to all contact points, including in between interventions	Fails to perform hand hygiene prior to patient contact or at any other intervention point
Introduces self to the patient and/or family professionally	Introduces self to patient and family, displays friendly, professional behavior at all times	Introduces self to patient and family in a professional manner	Fails to introduce self to patient and/or family, OR fails to introduce self professionally
Identifies the patient using a minimum of 2 patient identifiers	Identifies patient using 2 identifiers and explains reasoning to patient briefly	Identifies patient using 2 patient identifiers	Fails to identify patient prior to intervening
Prioritizes tasks to ensure most important tasks are completed first	Prioritizes all tasks appropriately, assists others with staying on task when necessary	Prioritizes most tasks appropriately, self-corrects when needed	Fails to prioritize tasks by most urgent needs (fails to place oxygen before notifying MD, for example)
Performs all tasks in an efficient and competent manner	Performs all tasks efficiently and competently, provides coaching to others when necessary	Works efficiently with minimal delays in providing interventions	Fails to work efficiently, makes critical errors that delay providing interventions
Specific Objectives			
Assesses patient and initiates therapeutic interventions	Meets Standards, AND Identifies need to assess for a Pulmonary Embolus	Assesses HR, RR, BP, SpO_2, Chest Pain, auscultates, attains chief complain and general patient appearance AND recognizes abnormal vital signs AND initiates O_2 therapy at a minimum of 2 L/min NC AND identifies possible cause of distress as a PE	Fails to meet one or more of the Standards

Learner Objectives	Pass		Needs Improvement
	Exceeds Standards	Meets Standards	Below Standards
Manages patient status appropriately		**Assesses need for nebulizer treatment AND gathers equipment necessary for an ABG and EKG AND correctly obtain blood sample and EKG rhythm strip**	Fails to meet one or more of the Standards
Analyzes and treats	Meets Standards, AND Correctly interpets EKG as normal AND requests anticoagulant therapy	Correctly interprets ABG as respiratory acidosis AND notifies MD of findings and patient condition AND documents interventions and patient status	Fails to meet one or more of the Standards

Other Comments for Student:

Evaluator: ______________________________

Student Name:

Personal Reflection

1. Write a SOAP note that summarizes the simulation.

2. List at least 3 things you've learned during this simulation.

3. A post-operative cholecystectomy patient develops sudden shortness of breath, and pleuritic chest pain. What is the most appropriate initial treatment?

   A. V/Q scan
   B. Supplemental oxygen
   C. Hemolytic therapy
   D. Thrombectomy

4. Which of the following are considered appropriate for treatment of a symptomatic pulmonary embolism?

   I. Heparin therapy
   II. Oxygen therapy
   III. Corticosteroids
   IV. Vasodilator

   A. I only
   B. I and II only
   C. II and IV only
   D. I, II, III, and IV

5. A clot that travels to the pulmonary trunk, getting caught at the bifurcation (at least partially blocking both the right and left pulmonary arteries) is known as what?

   A. Westermark sign
   B. Hamptom hump
   C. Saddle embolus
   D. Deep vein thrombosis

Further Reflection

6. Patients experiencing a pulmonary embolism may or may not have an abnormal PaO_2. Either way these patients may be hypoxemic and hypercapneic. How does this affect the alveolar-arterial oxygen tension gradient? Explain.

7. Develop a preventative plan that could be implemented in a healthcare facility that experiences a high volume of pulmonary emboli.

8. Deep vein thrombosis (DVT) accounts for a major percentage of all pulmonary emboli. What is a deep vein thrombosis? What causes it? What are the associated symptoms of a DVT?

PERFORMANCE CHECKLIST

Student Name: ______________________ Date Performed: ______________________

Learner Objectives	Pass		Needs Improvement
	Exceeds Standards	**Meets Standards**	**Below Standards**
General Objectives			
Performs hand hygiene at all appropriate intervention points	Intervenes and reminds others of need for PPE and hand hygiene	Washes hands prior to all contact points, including in between interventions	Fails to perform hand hygiene prior to patient contact or at any other intervention point
Introduces self to the patient and/or family professionally	Introduces self to patient and family, displays friendly, professional behavior at all times	Introduces self to patient and family in a professional manner	Fails to introduce self to patient and/or family, OR fails to introduce self professionally
Identifies the patient using a minimum of 2 patient identifiers	Identifies patient using 2 identifiers and explains reasoning to patient briefly	Identifies patient using 2 patient identifiers	Fails to identify patient prior to intervening
Prioritizes tasks to ensure most important tasks are completed first	Prioritizes all tasks appropriately, assists others with staying on task when necessary	Prioritizes most tasks appropriately, self-corrects when needed	Fails to prioritize tasks by most urgent needs (fails to place oxygen before notifying MD, for example)
Performs all tasks in an efficient and competent manner	Performs all tasks efficiently and competently, provides coaching to others when necessary	Works efficiently with minimal delays in providing interventions	Fails to work efficiently, makes critical errors that delay providing interventions
Specific Objectives			
Systematically assesses the patient after unplanned extubation	Meets Standards AND performs the assessment using a well-defined, targeted approach	Assesses patient with a systematic approach, including HR, RR, SpO_2 AND auscultates over larynx and lung fields AND has patient say something	Fails to meet one or more of the Standards
Initiates appropriate therapeutic interventions	Places patient on cool aerosol with minimal O_2 AND communicates with bedside RN to ensure close monitoring of patient	Places pt on minimum of 2 L/min Nasal Cannula via bubble humidifier	Fails to provide support OR fails to provide adequate support (to include some O_2 administration AND cool humidity)

Learner Objectives	Pass		Needs Improvement
	Exceeds Standards	Meets Standards	Below Standards
Recognizes signs and symptoms of post-extubation stridor	Recognizes potential signs and symptoms of post-extubation stridor within 1 minute AND auscultates larynx and lung fields AND notes change in HR, RR, BP, SpO_2	Recognizes potential signs and symptoms of post-extubation stridor within 2 minutes AND auscultates larynx and lung fields AND notes change in at least 2 of HR, RR, BP, SpO_2	Fails to recognize potential signs and symptoms of post-extubation stridor within 2 minutes OR fails to auscultate or assess patient adequately
Provides appropriate interventions for post-extubation stridor	Meets Standards, AND Vocalizes other possible therapies, including Heliox, reintubation, or additional racemic epinephrine dosage	Administers Racemic Epinephrine by small volume nebulizers after discussing with physician, and is able to give strength and dose AND reassesses patient after treatment	Fails to meet one or more of the Standards

Other Comments for Student:

Evaluator: ______________________________

Student Worksheet

1.14 Acacia Trinidad

by Scot Jones

Student Name:

Personal Reflection

1. Write a SOAP note that summarizes the simulation.

2. List at least 3 things you've learned during this simulation.

3. A 56-year old female, status post exploratory laparotomy , was being washed by the medical team, and her endotracheal tube was accidentally pulled out several centimeters. Which of the following is the best initial action for the Respiratory Practitioner to take?

   A. Pull the ET Tube the rest of the way out and prepare immediately for reintubation
   B. Insert ET Tube back to original charted lip marking and monitor closely
   C. Verify ET Tube placement using $ETCO_2$, chest rise, auscultation, and condensation in tube
   D. Draw a stat ABG and ensure respiratory sufficiency

4. After extubating a patient, you hear a musical tone over the upper airway. The patient is showing some accessory muscle use and is unable to speak in more than a few words. SpO_2 is reading 78% with a good waveform. Which of the following are appropriate responses?

   I. Administer 80% Helium / 20% Oxygen
   II. Administer 80% Oxygen / 20% Helium
   III. Administer Racemic epinephrine 2.25% via SVN
   IV. Place patient in reverse trendelenburg position

   A. I and III
   B. II and III
   C. II and IV
   D. I, III, and IV

Further Reflection

5. An 80-year old female has been intubated with a head bleed (Subdural Hematoma) after falling in her bathroom. She has been intubated and on a ventilator for 4 days now. The family has made the decision to change her code status to "Do Not Resuscitate." Later that day the patient is inadvertently extubated during a CXR. Her HR begins to drop and she is apneic. What should the medical team do at this time? Why?

6. What criteria should be used in determining whether to reintubate a patient or not?

7. List a minimum of 4 strategies that could be used to prevent inadvertent extubations.

PERFORMANCE CHECKLIST

Student Name: ______________________ Date Performed: ______________________

Learner Objectives	Pass		Needs Improvement
	Exceeds Standards	**Meets Standards**	**Below Standards**
General Objectives			
Performs hand hygiene at all appropriate intervention points	Intervenes and reminds others of need for PPE and hand hygiene	Washes hands prior to all contact points, including in between interventions	Fails to perform hand hygiene prior to patient contact or at any other intervention point
Introduces self to the patient and/or family professionally	Introduces self to patient and family, displays friendly, professional behavior at all times	Introduces self to patient and family in a professional manner	Fails to introduce self to patient and/or family, OR fails to introduce self professionally
Identifies the patient using a minimum of 2 patient identifiers	Identifies patient using 2 identifiers and explains reasoning to patient briefly	Identifies patient using 2 patient identifiers	Fails to identify patient prior to intervening
Prioritizes tasks to ensure most important tasks are completed first	Prioritizes all tasks appropriately, assists others with staying on task when necessary	Prioritizes most tasks appropriately, self-corrects when needed	Fails to prioritize tasks by most urgent needs (fails to place oxygen before notifying MD, for example)
Performs all tasks in an efficient and competent manner	Performs all tasks efficiently and competently, provides coaching to others when necessary	Works efficiently with minimal delays in providing interventions	Fails to work efficiently, makes critical errors that delay providing interventions
Specific Objectives			
Assesses patient using systematic approach for shortness of breath	Meets Standards, AND Assessment is well-targeted and systematic AND assesses for chest pain using pain scale	Discusses plan to assess with patient, auscultates all major lung fields, verifies vitals including HR, RR, BP, SpO_2, asks about SOB and for relevant past medical history	Fails to meet one or more of the Standards

Learner Objectives	Pass		Needs Improvement
	Exceeds Standards	Meets Standards	Below Standards
Initiates appropriate oxygen delivery device with appropriate flowrate and places on patient correctly	Meets Standards, AND Makes particular note of patient's SOB and RR which may require a high flow devices. Notes that a higher F_IO_2 could be appropriate, but should be considered witha tandem flow set-up	Initiates O_2 therapy within 1 minute of noting SpO_2, utilizing either Nasal Cannula (2- 3L/min) OR Nasal Cannula with bubble humidifier (4-6* L/min) OR Venti >30% at appropriate flow OR other appropriate device as indicated by instructor. Verifies acceptable improvement in $SpO_2 > 93\%$	Fails to meet one or more of the Standards
Reports on patient status to physician and recommends therapeutic interventions	Meets Standards, AND Independently recommends SABA SVN with correct dosage	Provides brief but relevant report to MD to include pertinent assessment (breath sounds, vitals, history) And informs MD about O_2 therapy AND recommends SABA SVN with correct dosage with minimal prompting by MD	Fails to meet one or more of the Standards
Administers nebulized SABA and assesses patient	Meets Standards, AND Performs exceptional instruction and technique	Collects drug, re-verifies pt identity (or uses barcode system if appropriate) AND administers SABA via SVN using correct instruction and technique AND assesses pt before, during, and after tx	Fails to meet one or more of the Standards
Optional: Dual Flow (Tandem) set up to meet high flow needs with varying SpO_2	Independently identifies need for tandem (see above)	With prompting by MD that uses terms like "varying SpO_2" and "high inspiratory flow need" student recognizes need to initiate tandem OR or is prompted to initiate AND correctly assembles and initiates dual flow (Tandem) set up	Fails to show understanding of need for tandem (dual flow) set-up despite instruction to do so

*Some texts allow for no humidity with a NC at 4 L/min, so this range is at instructor's discretion.

Other Comments for Student:

Evaluator: ______________________________

Student Worksheet

1.15 Sue Monas

by Scot Jones

Student Name:

Personal Reflection

1. Write a SOAP note that summarizes the simulation.

2. List at least 3 things you've learned during this simulation.

NBRC Preparation

3. A patient appears to be in distress with an SpO_2 of 86% and accessory muscle use. Currently he is on a 50% venti mask running at 12 L/min. His RR is 30/min, with good lung expansion noted. Of the following, which is the best choice?

   A. Maintain patient on current therapy and monitor closely
   B. Increase flow to 14 L/min
   C. Run another venti mask in tandem with the current one, running each at 12 L/min and 50%
   D. Ask for palliative care to come visit the patient

4. A 74-year old male has been admitted with a right upper lobe pneumonia. He is currently on a nasal cannula running at 2 L/min. He has a history of coronary artery disease, hypertension, and peripheral vascular disease. His SpO_2 is currently 84% with a plethysmograph that is erratic. He denies being short of breath. Which of the following should the RCP recommend?

   A. Correlate the pulse oximetry reading with an arterial blood gas
   B. Discontinue the pulse oximeter as it is ineffective in patients with peripheral vascular disease
   C. Clean the pulse oximeter thoroughly with an alcohol prep pad and reapply to the patient
   D. Intubate the patient and place on mechanical ventilation

Further Reflection

5. List the three types of pneumonias (by organism type), and for each provide the general category of treatment needed.

6. During report you note that the Respiratory Therapist says that a patient is suspected of having a pneumonia. What clinical information would support this suspicion? Be specific.

PERFORMANCE CHECKLIST

Student Name: ____________________ Date Performed: ____________________

Learner Objectives	Pass		Needs Improvement
	Exceeds Standards	**Meets Standards**	**Below Standards**
General Objectives			
Performs hand hygiene at all appropriate intervention points	Intervenes and reminds others of need for PPE and hand hygiene	Washes hands prior to all contact points, including in between interventions	Fails to perform hand hygiene prior to patient contact or at any other intervention point
Introduces self to the patient and/ or family professionally	Introduces self to patient and family, displays friendly, professional behavior at all times	Introduces self to patient and family in a professional manner	Fails to introduce self to patient and/ or family, OR fails to introduce self professionally
Identifies the patient using a minimum of 2 patient identifiers	Identifies patient using 2 identifiers and explains reasoning to patient briefly	Identifies patient using 2 patient identifiers	Fails to identify patient prior to intervening
Prioritizes tasks to ensure most important tasks are completed first	Prioritizes all tasks appropriately, assists others with staying on task when necessary	Prioritizes most tasks appropriately, self-corrects when needed	Fails to prioritize tasks by most urgent needs (fails to place oxygen before notifying MD, for example)
Performs all tasks in an efficient and competent manner	Performs all tasks efficiently and competently, provides coaching to others when necessary	Works efficiently with minimal delays in providing interventions	Fails to work efficiently, makes critical errors that delay providing interventions
Specific Objectives			
Performs initial patient assessment and recognizes abnormal signs and symptoms	Meets Standards, AND Verbalizes tension pneumothorax as potential cause of distress	Performs systematic patient assessment AND identifies hypoxemia, unequal chest wall movement, SOB, tachypnea AND requests CXR, EKG, and ABG AND initiates O_2 therapy AND notifies MD of findings AND initiates O_2 therapy	Fails to meet one or more of the Standards

Learner Objectives	Pass		Needs Improvement
	Exceeds Standards	Meets Standards	Below Standards
Correctly interprets test results and prepares for corrective measures	Meets Standards, AND Notifies MD, making specific recommendation for needle decompression and/or chest tube insertion	Identifies tension pneumothorax on CXR and/or through signs and symptoms AND correctly interprets ABG values (respiratory acidosis) and correctly interprets EKG rhythm as sinus tachycardia AND requests order for corrective measures	Failed to meet one or more of the Standards
Evaluates patient's response to interventions		Evaluates patient's response to interventions	Fails to evaluate patient's response to interventions
Notifies physician of patient's condition	Notifies physician of patient's condition using professional language AND provides very succinct, relevant details	Notifies physician of condition using professional language and covers all key aspects	Fails to notify physician OR neglects to mention important aspects

Other Comments for Student:

Evaluator: ______________________________

Student Worksheet

1.16 Jay St. Clair

by Sherry Whiteman

Student Name:

Personal Reflection

1. Write a SOAP note that summarizes the simulation.

2. List at least 3 things you've learned during this simulation.

3. A patient with asthma and chronic bronchitis experiences sudden onset of shortness of breath, hypotension, tachycardia, and diminished breath sounds on the left side. Of the following which is the most likely cause?

   A. Acute exacerbation of COPD
   B. Primary pneumothorax
   C. Bronchiectasis
   D. Secondary pneumothorax

4. A patient seen in the emergency department for a spontaneous pneumothorax is awaiting discharge. Which criteria must be met for the patient to be released from the hospital?

   I. Specialized testing for a bronchopleural fistula
   II. Primary spontaneous pneumothorax has been alleviated by simple aspiration
   III. Stable chest radiograph four hours post-aspiration procedure
   IV. Anterior chest tube connected to suction, with home education

   A. I and III
   B. II and III
   C. II and IV
   D. I, II, III, and IV

Further Reflection

5. Describe the effect of an untreated pneumothorax on CPR outcomes.

6. Differentiate between a primary and secondary spontaneous pneumothorax.

PERFORMANCE CHECKLIST (PATIENT 1)

Student Name: ______________________ Date Performed: ______________________

Learner Objectives	Pass		Needs Improvement
	Exceeds Standards	**Meets Standards**	**Below Standards**
General Objectives			
Performs hand hygiene at all appropriate intervention points	Intervenes and reminds others of need for PPE and hand hygiene	Washes hands prior to all contact points, including in between interventions	Fails to perform hand hygiene prior to patient contact or at any other intervention point
Introduces self to the patient and/or family professionally	Introduces self to patient and family, displays friendly, professional behavior at all times	Introduces self to patient and family in a professional manner	Fails to introduce self to patient and/or family, OR fails to introduce self professionally
Identifies the patient using a minimum of 2 patient identifiers	Identifies patient using 2 identifiers and explains reasoning to patient briefly	Identifies patient using 2 patient identifiers	Fails to identify patient prior to intervening
Prioritizes tasks to ensure most important tasks are completed first	Prioritizes all tasks appropriately, assists others with staying on task when necessary	Prioritizes most tasks appropriately, self-corrects when needed	Fails to prioritize tasks by most urgent needs (fails to place oxygen before notifying MD, for example)
Performs all tasks in an efficient and competent manner	Performs all tasks efficiently and competently, provides coaching to others when necessary	Works efficiently with minimal delays in providing interventions	Fails to work efficiently, makes critical errors that delay providing interventions
Specific Objectives			
Assesses the patient and recognizes thermal injury to the upper airway	Meets Standards, AND Notes ALL of the signs and symptoms	Recognizes thermal injury by noting MOST of the following: disclosure of smoke inhalation, black soot around mouth and nose, productive cough with coal-colored sputum, wheezing/stridor AND direct visualization of upper airway inflammation	Fails to meet one or more of the Standards

Learner Objectives	Pass		Needs Improvement
	Exceeds Standards	Meets Standards	Below Standards
Recognizes the need for and prepares for rapid sequence intubation	Meets Standards, AND Recommends appropriate drugs	Recognizes the need for rapid sequence intubation AND notifies physician AND prepares for RSI by setting up suction, pre-oxygenating, selecting proper airway, positioning patient, and monitoring patient AND appropriately assesses artificial airway placement AND places patient on ventilator or provides manual ventilation	Fails to meet one or more of the Standards
Responds to high likelihood of carbon monoxide positioning by providing and/or recommending appropriate therapeutic interventions	Meets Standards, AND Specifically notes high risk of CO poisoning despite high SpO2 AND recommends possibility of Hyperbaric Oxygen Therapy (with or without recommended settings) AND may recommend co-oximetry for carboxyhemoglobin lelves	Provides highest FIO_2 possible (via ventilator or Bag/Mask) while providing ventilations. Student may or may not make specific mention of hyperbarics and need for co-oximetry but does mention possibility of CO poisoning	Fails to meet one or more of the Standards
Notifies physician of patient's condition and documents interventions	Meets Standards, AND Notification of physician is very concise	Notifies physician of events leading up to intervention, makes appropriate recommendations, and documents all interventions	Fails to meet one or more of the Standards

Other Comments for Student:

Evaluator: ______________________________

Student Worksheet

1.17 M. Traige

by Janice Dunaway

Student Name:

Personal Reflection

1. Write a SOAP note that summarizes the simulation.

2. List at least 3 things you've learned during this simulation.

3. All of the following are considered a fire risk inside a hyperbaric oxygen chamber, except:

   A. Petroleum jelly (like Vaseline)
   B. Alcohol-based disinfectants
   C. 100% cotton clothing
   D. Cell phone

4. A 45-year old male was rescued from a house fire and transported to the ED. He was intubated to protect his airway and was placed on mechanical ventilation. He was reported to be 6 feet tall, and weighs approximately 300 lb. Which of the following ventilator settings would be the best choice for this patient?

   A. SIMV, Rate 12, VT 650 mL, O_2 100%
   B. V-A/C, Rate 16, VT 850 mL, O_2 100%
   C. P-A/C, Rate 10, VT 950 mL, O_2 100%
   D. CPAP 10 cmH_2O, O_2 80%

5. Which of the following would be the best choice for supplying oxygen to a patient following smoke inhalation?

   A. Nasal cannula at 6 L/min
   B. 40% Venturi mask
   C. Non-rebreathing mask running at about 12 L/min
   D. Cool mist aerosol mask using a large volume nebulizer at 100%

Further Reflection

6. List some of the signs of thermal injury to the glottis, larynx, and vocal cords.

7. Discuss the effect abnormal hemoglobins, like carboxyhemoglobin and methemoglobin, have on oxygenation (don't just say they decrease oxygenation - give a well thought out answer that takes the physiology into account).

8. List at least three criteria for the use of hyperbaric oxygen therapy in carbon monoxide poisoning.

9. While Hyperbaric Oxygen Therapy (HBOT) is life-saving for some people, and is widely used in wound healing, there are some complications we need to be aware of. List a minimum of 3 hazards related to HBOT.

PERFORMANCE CHECKLIST

Student Name: ____________________ Date Performed: ____________________

Learner Objectives	Pass		Needs Improvement
	Exceeds Standards	Meets Standards	Below Standards
General Objectives			
Performs hand hygiene at all appropriate intervention points	Intervenes and reminds others of need for PPE and hand hygiene	Washes hands prior to all contact points, including in between interventions	Fails to perform hand hygiene prior to patient contact or at any other intervention point
Introduces self to the patient and/or family professionally	Introduces self to patient and family, displays friendly, professional behavior at all times	Introduces self to patient and family in a professional manner	Fails to introduce self to patient and/or family, OR fails to introduce self professionally
Identifies the patient using a minimum of 2 patient identifiers	Identifies patient using 2 identifiers and explains reasoning to patient briefly	Identifies patient using 2 patient identifiers	Fails to identify patient prior to intervening
Prioritizes tasks to ensure most important tasks are completed first	Prioritizes all tasks appropriately, assists others with staying on task when necessary	Prioritizes most tasks appropriately, self-corrects when needed	Fails to prioritize tasks by most urgent needs (fails to place oxygen before notifying MD, for example)
Performs all tasks in an efficient and competent manner	Performs all tasks efficiently and competently, provides coaching to others when necessary	Works efficiently with minimal delays in providing interventions	Fails to work efficiently, makes critical errors that delay providing interventions
Specific Objectives			
Systematically assesses the patient in distress	Meets Standards, AND Palpates for subcutaneous emphysema AND BOTH examines inner cannula AND inserts suctions catheter into the tracheostomy, identifying concern with airway patency quickly	Quickly but systematically assesses the patient in distress which includes vital signs AND auscultation AND verification of airway patency	Fails to meet one or more of the Standards

Learner Objectives	Pass		Needs Improvement
	Exceeds Standards	Meets Standards	Below Standards
Removes artificial airway and begins manual resuscitation	Removes artificial airway within 2 minutes of initial entry into room AND begins to provide bag/mask ventilation with O_2 by either occluding mouth and bagging via stoma (preferably with pediatric mask) OR by occluding stoma and bagging by mouth (**unless total laryngectomy scenario**)	Removes artificial airway within 3 minutes of initial entry into room AND begins to provide bag/mask ventilation with O_2 by either occluding mouth and bagging via stoma (preferably with pediatric mask) OR by occluding stoma and bagging by mouth (**unless total laryngectomy scenario**)	Fails to remove artificial airway within 3 minutes of initial entry into room OR fails to begin bag/mask ventilating appropriately
Re-establishes patent airway	Re-establishes airway by confidently either: inserting small ET Tube into stoma (#6.0) OR inserting new tracheostomy tube OR intubating orally (**unless total laryngectomy scenario**)	Continues to provide manual ventilation to patient while seeking physician input. Eventually re-establishes airway by either inserting small ET Tube into stoma (#6.0) OR inserting new tracheostomy tube OR intubating orally (**unless total laryngectomy scenario**)	Fails to provide adequate ventilation OR fails to re-establish patency of airway by either seeking assistance from physician AND providing a plan OR inserting a new airway
Confirms placement of patent airway	Immediately confirms placement of airway by using $ETCO_2$, Chest Rise, Auscultation and by passing suction catheter down airway. IF TRACH identifies immediately that airway is not patent	Confirms placement by minimally using $ETCO_2$ detector, chest rise, and auscultation. IF TRACH identifies immediately that airway is not patent	Fails to confirm placement of new airway OR fails to recognize airway is still not patent

Other Comments for Student:

Evaluator: ______________________

Student Worksheet

1.18 Phillip Floyd

by Scot Jones

Student Name:

Personal Reflection

1. Write a SOAP note that summarizes the simulation.

2. List at least 3 things you've learned during this simulation.

3. The Respiratory Care Practitioner is working in the Intensive Care Unit and receives a patient from the OR who has had a surgical tracheostomy placed following a total laryngectomy. A short while later the patient is inadvertently decannulated during a bath. His SpO_2 is reading 80%. Which of the following steps should be performed first?

    A. Monitor the patient closely and obtain an ABG
    B. Intubate patient via the mouth immediately
    C. Provide manual ventilation by a pediatric mask over the stoma, and then insert ET Tube gently into stoma and inflate cuff
    D. Insert spare tracheostomy of equal size into the stoma and verify placement

4. A new tracheostomy patient is arriving in the unit where the Respiratory Care Practitioner is working. The RCP should have all of the following available at the bedside, EXCEPT:

    A. Manual resuscitation bag with mask
    B. Tracheostomy tube one size larger than the one placed
    C. Tracheostomy tube one size smaller than the one placed
    D. Obturator

5. Which of the following is least likely to cause subcutaneous emphysema (crepitus)?

    A. Tracheotomy tube lodged in the soft tissue around the stoma
    B. Pneumothorax following subclavian central line placement
    C. Transudative pleural effusion related to cardiac failure
    D. The presence of an infection, like fournier gangrene

Further Reflection

6. Fill in the following table:

Type	Typical Reasons for being placed	How to Ventilate in an Emergency	Options for replacing if decannulated
Tracheostomy			
Total Laryngectomy			

7. You are asked to verify the patency of a tracheostomy that is in place. List at least 3 ways you could do this at the bedside.

PERFORMANCE CHECKLIST

Student Name: ______________________ Date Performed: ______________________

Learner Objectives	Pass		Needs Improvement
	Exceeds Standards	Meets Standards	Below Standards
General Objectives			
Performs hand hygiene at all appropriate intervention points	Intervenes and reminds others of need for PPE and hand hygiene	Washes hands prior to all contact points, including in between interventions	Fails to perform hand hygiene prior to patient contact or at any other intervention point
Introduces self to the patient and/or family professionally	Introduces self to patient and family, displays friendly, professional behavior at all times	Introduces self to patient and family in a professional manner	Fails to introduce self to patient and/or family, OR fails to introduce self professionally
Identifies the patient using a minimum of 2 patient identifiers	Identifies patient using 2 identifiers and explains reasoning to patient briefly	Identifies patient using 2 patient identifiers	Fails to identify patient prior to intervening
Prioritizes tasks to ensure most important tasks are completed first	Prioritizes all tasks appropriately, assists others with staying on task when necessary	Prioritizes most tasks appropriately, self-corrects when needed	Fails to prioritize tasks by most urgent needs (fails to place oxygen before notifying MD, for example)
Performs all tasks in an efficient and competent manner	Performs all tasks efficiently and competently, provides coaching to others when necessary	Works efficiently with minimal delays in providing interventions	Fails to work efficiently, makes critical errors that delay providing interventions
Specific Objectives			
Initiates mechanical ventilation	Performs ventilator set-up and sets appropriate mode and settings for patient pathophysiology AND performs ventilator monitoring AND determines readiness for lung recruitment (evidenced by BP > 90/60, HR within normal limits)	Performs ventilator set-up and sets appropriate mode and settings for patient pathophysiology AND performs ventilator monitoring and determines basic need for lung recruitment OR contacts MD for order to perform recruitment	Fails to perform ventilator set-up OR sets inappropriate initial settings OR does not perform ventilator monitoring OR fails to calls physician

Learner Objectives	Pass		Needs Improvement
	Exceeds Standards	Meets Standards	Below Standards
Performs lung recruitment	Initiates lung recruitment maneuver using proper technique AND notifies MD/RN prior to initiation AND monitors patient's hemodynamic status during procedure AND verbalizes need to stop if patient becomes unstable AND initiates optimal PEEP settings	Initiates lung recruitment maneuver using proper technique AND monitors patient's hemodynamic status during procedure AND identifies patient's optimal PEEP AND initiates optimal PEEP settings	Fails to perform lung recruitment maneuver using proper technique OR fails to monitor patient's hemodynamic status during procedure OR fails to identify optimal PEEP settings
Closely monitors patient	Evaluates patient's response to recruitment maneuver AND identifies at least 2 ways to determine effectiveness of maneuver AND verbalizes (when asked) 2 possible hazards to monitor during and after maneuver AND identifies (when asked) 2 contraindications to recruitment maneuvers AND notifies physician of patient's condition and new settings AND documents interventions and patient's status	Evaluates patient's response to recruitment maneuver AND identifies at least 2 ways to determine effectiveness of maneuver AND notifies physician of patient's condition and new settings AND documents interventions and patient's status	Fails to evaluate patient's response to recruitment maneuver OR fails to identify ways to determine effectiveness of maneuver OR fails to notify physician of patient's condition OR fails to document interventions and patient's status

Other Comments for Student:

Evaluator: ______________________________

Student Worksheet

1.19 Sadie Stark

by Sherry Whiteman

Student Name:

Personal Reflection

1. Write a SOAP note that summarizes the simulation.

2. List at least 3 things you've learned during this simulation.

3. When using a pressure-volume curve to provide lung protective ventilation, the PEEP should be set at:

   A. 5 cm H_2O above subambient pressure
   B. 1-2 cm H_2O above the Upper Inflection Point
   C. 5 cm H_2O below subambient pressure
   D. 1-2 cm H_2O above the Lower Infection Point

4. Which of the following are potential causes of Pulseless Electrical Activity?
   I. Thrombosis
   II. Hypothermia
   III. Toxoplasmosis
   IV. Histoplasmosis

   A. I only
   B. III only
   C. I and II only
   D. II and IV only

5. A patient is experiencing pulseless electrical activity (PEA) and cardiopulmonary resuscitation is in progress. The first 2 minutes of CPR have been completed and PEA persists, so CPR is resumed. What is the next BEST intervention?

   A. Synchronized cardioversion
   B. Defibrillation
   C. Atropine administration
   D. Epinephrine administration

Further Reflection

6. As you participate in physician rounding on a patient who is status post CABG, the physician states that the patient has active bleeding inside the thoracic cavity. He turns to you, as the Respiratory Therapist, and asks for recommendations related to the ventilator. What do you suggest?

7. About 24-hours after completion of a quadruple bypass, a patient begins to exhibit the following rhythm on the monitor. Identify the rhythm, the likely cause, and the correct treatment.

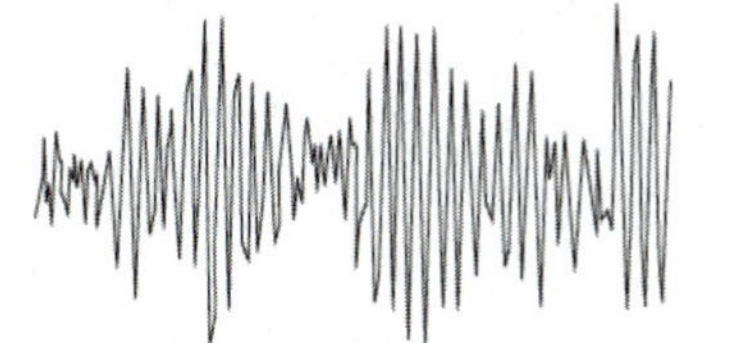

8. A patient is status post CABG x2 - about 12 hours ago. The patient has been exhibiting signs of decreased cardiac output and stroke volume, as well as hypotension and JVD. During your patient-ventilator assessment, you note that the patient appears quite pale. There is no palpable pulse and you note the following rhythm:

   A. What should you do first?

   B. Identify this rhythm.

   C. What is the most likely cause of this rhythm?

   D. How should this rhythm be treated?

PERFORMANCE CHECKLIST

Student Name: ______________________ Date Performed: ______________________

Learner Objectives	Pass		Needs Improvement
	Exceeds Standards	Meets Standards	Below Standards
General Objectives			
Performs hand hygiene at all appropriate intervention points	Intervenes and reminds others of need for PPE and hand hygiene	Washes hands prior to all contact points, including in between interventions	Fails to perform hand hygiene prior to patient contact or at any other intervention point
Introduces self to the patient and/or family professionally	Introduces self to patient and family, displays friendly, professional behavior at all times	Introduces self to patient and family in a professional manner	Fails to introduce self to patient and/or family, OR fails to introduce self professionally
Identifies the patient using a minimum of 2 patient identifiers	Identifies patient using 2 identifiers and explains reasoning to patient briefly	Identifies patient using 2 patient identifiers	Fails to identify patient prior to intervening
Prioritizes tasks to ensure most important tasks are completed first	Prioritizes all tasks appropriately, assists others with staying on task when necessary	Prioritizes most tasks appropriately, self-corrects when needed	Fails to prioritize tasks by most urgent needs (fails to place oxygen before notifying MD, for example)
Performs all tasks in an efficient and competent manner	Performs all tasks efficiently and competently, provides coaching to others when necessary	Works efficiently with minimal delays in providing interventions	Fails to work efficiently, makes critical errors that delay providing interventions
Specific Objectives			
Rapidly and systematically assesses the patient	Immediately recognizes need to assess patient, and performs very targeted brief systematic assessment, including Circulation, Airway, Breathing (per BLS guidelines), as well as checking SpO_2 and asking nurse pertinent questions	Immediately recognizes need to assess patient, systematically assessing vital signs, checking SpO_2, and asking the patient and nurse pertinent questions	Fails to recognize need to immediately assess patient OR fails to assess vital signs or SpO_2 OR fails to ask patient/nurse pertinent questions
Recognizes respiratory depression and identifies over-medication as the most likely cause	Immediately recognizes respiratory depression and identifies over-medication as most likely cause AND immediately begins to initiate action steps to support patient's status	Recognizes and verbalizes probability of respiratory depression and begins to initiate action steps to support patient's status	Fails to recognize respiratory depression OR fails to begin to initiate action steps to support patient's status

Learner Objectives	Pass		Needs Improvement
	Exceeds Standards	Meets Standards	Below Standards
Provides appropriate airway management and ventilatory support in context of respiratory depression	Positions patient optimally immediate following recognition of depression AND provides very good C:E technique with mask OR requests assistance in providing two-person airway management. Shows outstanding awareness of monitoring while managing airway.	Optimally places patient to open airway AND provides ventilation using good C:E technique with manual resuscitator and mask, monitoring for chest rise and improving SpO_2	Fails to position patient optimally OR fails to provide appropriate bag/mask ventilation using C:E technique OR fails to monitor patient once providing bag/mask ventilation
Recommends administration of reversal agent	Recommends administration of reversal agent AND continues to provide adequate ventilation until patient awakens AND monitors closely, nothing patient goes back into respiratory depression AND recommends administration of 2nd dose of reversal agent	Recommends administration of reversal agent AND continues to provide adequate ventilation until patient awakens AND monitors closely	Fails to recommend administration of reversal agent OR fails to provide adequate ventilation OR fails to monitor closely

Other Comments for Student:

Evaluator: ______________________________

Student Worksheet

by Scot Jones

Student Name:

Personal Reflection

1. Write a SOAP note that summarizes the simulation.

2. List at least 3 things you've learned during this simulation.

3. As a member of the rapid response team, The RCP is the first to arrive to a call. Upon arrival the patient, who is on room air, is noted to be diaphoretic, tachypneic, and tachycardic. SpO_2 is 93%. When asked about pain, he complains about constant chest pain. The first thing the RCP should do is:

    A. Begin chest compressions
    B. Notify the patient's physician
    C. Place the patient on 2 L/min Nasal Cannula
    D. Carefully observe the patient until the rest of the rapid response team arrives

4. During a rapid response call, a lethargic patient is noted to have a decreased respiratory rate of 6-8/minute. Her breathing is noted to be shallow. While investigating the cause for the depression in ventilation, the Respiratory Therapist should:

    A. Place an oropharyngeal airway (OPA)
    B. Provide manual breaths using a bag and mask, giving about one breath every 5-6 seconds
    C. Perform nasotracheal suctioning, and then give supplemental oxygen
    D. Intubate the patient and place on mechanical ventilation

5. During a rapid response call, a stuporous patient, has a decreased respiratory rate, SpO_2 86%, and the EKG rhythm on the portable monitor suggests the patient is in Sinus Tachycardia with brief runs of Ventricular Tachycardia. BP is 90/44. Respiratory Rate is 6-8 breaths/min and irregular. The Respiratory Therapist should:

    A. Place an oropharyngeal airway (OPA)
    B. Provide manual breaths using a bag and mask, giving about one breath every 5-6 seconds
    C. Perform nasotracheal suctioning, and then give supplemental oxygen
    D. Intubate the patient and place on mechanical ventilation

Further Reflection

6. As it relates to a rapid response call, explain what systematic assessment is. How is it different than how you would assess a patient at other times?

7. In your opinion, how do patients end up over-medicated for pain in the hospital? Is this preventable?